DISCLAIMER and COPYRIGHT

The reader should consult with their doctor in any matters relating to his/her health.

The information contained within this eBook is strictly for educational purposes. If you wish to apply ideas contained in this eBook, you are taking full responsibility for your actions. The author has made every effort to ensure the accuracy of the information within this book was correct at the time of publication. The author does not assume and hereby disclaims any liability to any party for any loss, damage, or disruption caused by errors or omissions, whether such errors or omissions result from accident, negligence, or any other cause. By reading onwards, you abolish the author of this eBook of all liability and accept the disclaimer and copyright terms and conditions.

Deep Tissue Massage

Jargon-Free Guide to Relieve Stress and Live Relaxed

By: M.S.D

CONTENTS

Disclaimer and Copyright

Introduction

Chapter 1: What Is Deep Tissue Massage Therapy?

Chapter 2: How It Works

Chapter 3: Benefits of Deep Tissue Massage

Chapter 4: How Deep Tissue Massage Therapy Helps

Chapter 5: Techniques and the Cost of Therapy

Chapter 6: Pros and Cons

Chapter 7: Treatment Options

Chapter 8: Before and After Results

Chapter 9: The Final Verdict

Author's Note

INTRODUCTION

You may have come across this book to know about deep tissue massage therapy and you have made the right choice. This is a self-help book that covers all that you need to know about deep tissue massage therapy in terms of how it can be beneficial to you.

Many people don't think much about their muscles and the underlying soft tissues until some pain, stiffness or tension arises, but there are also those who keep searching for help in aiding chronic muscle pain and tension as well as their postural problems. Most of us have felt a knot or discomfort at one time or another after our daily activities, workouts or leisure events. This can be treated with deep tissue massage therapy. You need to take care of the muscles, tendons, ligaments, bones and joints for your overall health and wellness.

Deep tissue massage therapy reaches out to the root of the problem in the core of the muscles that cause pain, tension, soreness and discomfort and it is therefore more beneficial than many other types of therapies-although it is often confused with other massage therapies such as Swedish massage. When recipients whom undergo treatment such as a full body massage for relaxation, a lot of the time they are told that it is deep tissue massage but many times it is not.

This type of massage is little known about therefore it may be in your best interest to know what it is, how it works, its benefits and cost, the techniques used and the precautions you need to be aware of among other considerations. This e-book is all about that and it takes you through what you need to know about deep tissue massage therapy and how it can help you overcome chronic pain, muscle tension, stiffness, soreness, rejuvenate the sore tissues and heal conditions in addition to promoting health and wellness.

The muscles are divided into layers and while many massage therapies address the top layers, only a few concentrate on the deeper soft tissues-this is where deep tissue massage theory shines. Deep tissue massage concentrates on the deeper layers to alleviate pain and tension while assisting the lymphatic system and blood circulatory system to rid the toxins contained in the tissues. Deep tissue massage therapy is both therapeutic and corrective. The therapist delivering the massage applies gentle strokes to allow the body to relax while pressing the muscles deeply in a systematic way to release pain, tension and toxins as well as in some cases correct postural problems. Read through and solidify your understanding of the therapeutic principles mentioned in this informative guide to ensure you relieve all your stresses and live a relaxed life-isolating all the chaos around you.

CHAPTER ONE

What is Deep Tissue Massage Therapy

Deep tissue massage therapy is a type of massage that is aimed at the deep muscle layers, specifically the soft tissues in the body and the connective tissue that surrounds the muscles, bones and joints known as fascia. Many people refer to full body massages- especially when it is administered for a long time- as deep tissue massage therapy but that may not necessarily be the case.

Deep tissue muscle therapy movements are slow while the pressure is deeply aimed at the areas feeling pain and tension. Some of these movements similarly compare to the ones used in classic massage therapy although with deep tissue massage, they are focused on the deep layers of muscles and the connective tissue. Deep tissue massage can help with chronic pain and muscle stress by relieving pain and tension of a stiff neck, upper and lower back pain, muscle tightness in the legs, IT band, hamstrings, biceps, quadriceps and soreness in the shoulders.

Our muscles tire from time to time which can affect the way we feel physically, emotionally and mentally. The muscles may form knots which trap toxins in the system. Bands of tissues can contract or grip onto muscles, joints, bones, tendons and ligaments causing postural imbalances and irregularities in our bodily functions. The bands can be gently pressed by a qualified therapist in order to break them down to release any areas they previously held and as a result the posture can be corrected.

When deep tissue massage is administered by a professional therapist, the knots are undone and the toxins are released into the body's excretion system. The recipient may not immediately feel relaxed when compared to other classic massage therapies, in fact mild pain, soreness and tenderness may be felt after the massage instead of relaxation. However, these symptoms typically fade away in a day or two after which the recipient should feel much better than before the massage was given. This gives any recipient of deep tissue massage therapy the reason to carry on with treatment especially if other therapies just don't seem to work.

You should not be afraid to go for a deep tissue massage treatment. Although this therapy is deeper and more intense on the body than other types of massage, it should not be excruciatingly painful. It is true that you may feel some degree of discomfort especially if your condition is severe, but the affected areas of the body can be worked on slowly over a long period of time and the treatment can still yield effective results. You need to establish your threshold of pain and pressure level of what you can tolerate to ensure optimal pressure is administered. If the condition of your muscles is mild, one session should be enough for you.

Executives who encounter stress-related work, office workers, people who have physically demanding jobs, IT and computer personnel, secretaries, writers, drivers, marathon runners and generally energetic people carrying out their daily functions of life can all be prone to knots, tension and stiffness in their muscles. Sitting for long hours at a desk or in front of a computer doing repetitive work or carrying, pulling and pushing loads without the proper technique and training can lead to postural problems. The neck, shoulders, upper and lower back, hamstring, biceps and quadriceps can tense up and become sore. Deep tissue massage can help unwind and heal the muscles, tendons, ligaments, bones and joints as well as diffuse any stress leading to rejuvenation of the whole body.

CHAPTER TWO

How it Works

When someone has muscle tensions or has suffered an injury, their muscles, tendons and ligaments can get painful and rigid bands or adhesions may form within the tissue. As a result, the adhesions can then block blood flow which then leads to pain, inflammation and limited mobility of the muscles or joints. The rigidness causes pain, stiffness and tension as in the case of sports injuries or injuries due to workouts, bodybuilding and sometimes even normal everyday activities. This can happen in any part of the body. Deep tissue massage therapy, when applied in such areas can break down the tissue scars and adhesions relieving pain and inflammation and restoring normal movement and proper blood flow.

Many things can cause muscles and the connective tissues to tighten and cause tension which can then lead to pain and stiffness.

These may include the following:

- Sports injuries and falls

- Overuse

- Limited mobility

- Whiplash

- Osteoarthritis pain

- Fibromyalgia

- Tennis elbow

- Repetitive strain injury like carpal tunnel syndrome

- Sciatica

Carpal tunnel syndrome and tennis elbow are conditions which can be caused by overusing muscles and performing repetitive tasks. As a result, muscle fibers may become tense and then shorten. Similar problems can occur with the connective tissue which line the muscles, bones and joints of the body. Scar tissue known as fibrosis may also form.

When the muscle fibers are stiff and tense, there is reduced blood flow to areas throughout the body since the toxins get held up in the tissues because the lymphatic system is unable to get rid of them fast enough which adds to congestion. This causes pain and soreness which calls upon deep tissue massage therapy as being the only option to have the waste products caused by the body's metabolism to be released and eliminated from the tissues altogether. The massage helps the shortened and hardened muscle fibers to get lengthened and softened while the adhesions are broken down and the tightened tissues and joints free up. After the massage, the muscle fibers are separated as they should normally be. This restores their elasticity and flexibility and any postural imbalances correct themselves as a result.

When the therapist massages the deep tissues in a gentle yet firm manner, the blood circulation improves and the muscles, tendons, ligaments, the connective tissue and joints loosen up and relax, making them move as they should. The scar tissue can be broken down or reduced with consistent deep tissue massaging. All these processes help to provide pain relief, release tension, correct posture and increase flexibility which ultimately aids in mobility. Direct and deep pressure on the affected areas coupled with massage oils, lotion or gel can be of great assistance for effective healing. During treatment, the muscles are first relaxed with gentle strokes before the therapist applies deep pressure. This is done in a systematic way so long-term effects can be achieved and sustained.

The therapist is careful and sensitive to affected areas while applying pressure. The pace at which deep tissue massage is performed is usually slower than that of other massage therapies in order to allow the therapist to understand the tissues and service them accordingly. The tension and "knots" found within the muscles are massaged with the utmost care to ensure that there is minimal-if any-pain on behalf of the recipient of the massage and also no strain on the part of the therapist either. To achieve lasting releases of toxins from the contractions and "knots", the recipient must remain relaxed and comfortable. On the other hand, the therapist has to be sensitive enough to understand the problematic areas and gently work them without upsetting the relaxation of the recipient otherwise the recipient's muscles can tighten due to pain or discomfort in which case the body's natural reflex actions can take over which will-once again-cause muscle contractions, defeating the purpose of treatment.

One session of deep tissue massage is not enough to allow you to thoroughly reap the benefits of therapy. You need to undergo massages consistently to experience the advantages associated with this therapy. If you are a beginner, it may be in your best interests to search for a certified professional therapist or ask for credible referrals from your physician, family or friends.

Typically, the treatment starts off by the having the therapist take your general medical history and perform an evaluation of your current state of wellbeing while asking you about the specific areas you want to be massaged for as well as if you have any extremely painful areas which should be avoided totally. You should work with your therapist to choose the pressure level which you are comfortable with. When in pain, breathing in deeply helps to discard any minor discomforts you may feel during the massage however, you should alert your therapist immediately if you feel any unbearable pain. Do not naturally assume the pain to be part of the process, convey any discomforts in full disclosure to your therapist. Communication between you and the therapist is very important to ensure you receive the treatment with its full potential and reap all the benefits, not add to your problems.

CHAPTER THREE

Benefits of Deep Tissue Massage

There are many benefits associated with deep tissue massage such as the following:

•Pain relief and management

•Reduces chronic muscle, tendon and ligament pain and tension

•Improves blood circulation and lymphatic circulation

•Lowers blood pressure

•Rehabilitates injured muscles

•Relieves stress

•Improves posture, flexibility and physical appearance

•Rids the body of toxins

Pain Relief and Management

Pain relief is one of the many benefits derived from deep tissue massage, although the effect may not be felt immediately. People who suffer from conditions such as osteoarthritis, fibromyalgia, tennis elbow and carpal tunnel syndrome can experience pain relief as a result of consistent deep tissue massage therapy. This therapy may be used as a treatment option to manage pain in similar conditions to the ones listed above as well-ask your therapist since they most likely have seen it all in their practise.

Reduces Chronic Pain, Tension and Stiffness

Deep tissue massage is said to be a more effective and an affordable way of treating chronic pain, tension and stiffness of the muscles, tendons, ligaments, fascia and joints when compared to certain specialized massages. It is known to be more effective than exercise, physical therapy and conventional medicine especially in treating conditions like osteoarthritis pain.

Improves Blood Circulation and Lymphatic Circulation

Clogged arteries and veins benefit from this massage tremendously. The blood circulation improves as a result of clearing the congestion in the body's pathways of flow. Oxygen-enriched blood containing essential nutrients is transported all over the body through its internal pathways which then works to relieve pain, soreness and inflammation in the affected areas which were previously susceptible to inadequate blood circulation. Muscle tension causes pain therefore, when the muscles are massaged, the tension is released and pain is alleviated as the end result. The toxins released from the tissues during the massage are then eliminated by the body's lymphatic system.

Lowers Blood Pressure

Deep tissue massage can also help to lower blood pressure since the stress and tension is relieved allowing the body's internal functions to sync and balance themselves. A 45 to 60 minute session is enough to lower blood pressure by a noticeable amount.

Rehabilitates Injured Muscles

When you receive deep tissue massage after suffering any muscle injuries whether it be a result of everyday activities, falls, workouts or playing sports, the toxins are carried away by the lymphatic system and the improved blood circulation and lymphatic circulation ultimately promotes the body's healing process. Deep tissue sports massages may help to rehabilitate injured muscles, tendons and ligaments for sports oriented individuals such as marathoners and the players of soccer, tennis, cricket, hockey and other sports. This variation of deep tissue massage caters to the active individuals and may also be used to supplement their sport by getting a thorough treatment as part of their training routine.

Relieves Stress

When your muscles, tendons and ligaments are stressed they cause pain-as you've learned so far. There are also people who suffer from chronic stress and its associated side effects which include headaches caused by constant tension, tense muscles and rigidness in shoulders-all of which can be relieved by implementing deep tissue massage therapy. 45-60 minutes of massage can reduce the stress hormonal levels and has the ability to trigger the body's natural feel-good hormones which aid in boosting your overall mood.

Reduces Scar Tissue

Deep tissue massage breaks down and reduces the scar tissue in the body due to better blood circulation and drainage that takes place within the body's lymphatic system. The increased range of motion and flexibility in the previously affected areas also makes it easier to further break down any scar tissue which may still be present. This relieves pain and stiffness caused by the scar tissue which may also finally disappear with consistent massage.

Improves Posture, Flexibility, Mobility and Physical Appearance

People with postural problems benefit greatly from this therapy.

CHAPTER FOUR

How Deep Tissue Massage Therapy Helps

Many things may cause muscles to become painfully stiff and tense. This is quite common in the neck, shoulders, and the upper and lower back. Work related activities can cause postural problems and overuse of muscles. Leisure activities such as sports, gardening, hiking or running may also be the culprit to these problems.

Whether you are a weekend jogger, a hiker or a professional athlete, you stand to gain a lot from a good sports massage which is similar to deep tissue massage. You will receive massages oriented at your specific needs depending on which parts of your body has been overused or stressed due to your specific sport. The therapy can be thought of-as well as prescribed-as part of your training regimen. It can also be administered to minimize recovery time after a recent injury and can be used for recovery in general after intense training.

The type of therapy you are given will depend on the area of the body that is affected and your daily habits which trigger such problems, whether it be a leisurely exercise or a professional sport. Remember to always communicate with your therapist to determine your tolerance level and establish a threshold for pain prior to the starting of your session.

Deep tissue massage therapy helps with the following:

•Lower back pain

•Rehabilitation of injuries such as stiff neck, whiplash, sports and fall injuries

•Tennis elbow

•Repetitive strain injuries like carpal tunnel syndrome

•Muscle tension or spasms in the legs, hamstrings, upper back, quadriceps

•Osteoarthritis pain

Lower Back Pain

People with lower back pain benefit a great deal from deep tissue massage. The massage therapist realigns the muscles together with the connective tissue during the massage process by pressing the spaces and gaps between the muscles deeply and firmly while simultaneously massaging the surrounding areas. This corrects any alignment issues and relieves stress restoring the natural form of your lower back.

The massage helps patients to recover from injuries such as whiplash, sports related, slips and falls and other injuries of similar aspects, faster than what would have been possible otherwise. This happens when the lymphatic system is triggered with deep and firm massage techniques to carry away the toxins from the injured muscle tissues which in return accelerates the healing process.

Tennis Elbow

People who develop tennis elbow whether it be a result of repetitive typing, working on computers or playing sports can greatly benefit from deep tissue massage therapy. The treatment can cure tennis elbow by realigning the elbow joint to its natural position as close as possible relieving pain and disability which was previously felt with the misalignment. The massage process requires a thorough knowledge and deep understanding of the muscles affected which is why you need to choose a professional therapist who is competent in the subject of matter.

Muscle tensions and spasms can arise while walking, playing sports and doing other active activities, especially if someone has not been active for a while. Any part of the body can get muscle tension and spasms but usually the hamstrings, neck, shoulders, back and legs are the typical victims. Massage can relieve contractions within these areas making you feel great afterwards. Do not be discouraged to get back to your usual routine after a long period of inactivity, deep tissue massage is there to help in case you feel any mild discomforts afterwards. However, ease into the activities you previously might have done swiftly to allow for your muscles to adapt to their previous nature. This will also ensure no further injury is sustained.

CHAPTER FIVE

Techniques and Cost of Therapy

Deep tissue massage is similar to physical therapy because of the involvement of the patient. Usually in massage therapy, the patient relaxes while the therapist performs massage. Some patients may even fall asleep due to the calming atmosphere and relaxation of the body. Often soft music is played to enhance the relaxation process. Deep tissue therapy shares some of the same characteristics however, it slightly differs. When deep tissue massage therapy is being administered, the patient may need to participate in activities such as deep breathing upon the therapist's requests to further aid in the loosening of contractions. It is advisable that the patient stays awake-yet still remain relaxed.

The main techniques used are as follows:

- •Active Motion

- •Passive Motion

- •Static Pressure

- •Negative Pressure

- •Muscle Capping

Active Motion

Active Motion involves flexing and stretching muscles as they are being worked on while the therapist strokes and presses them firmly. The client flexes the muscles in order for the fibers to spread, allowing the therapist to massage deeply in between these muscle fibers. This can take as long as 15 to 20 minutes or as little as 5 to 10 minutes for effectively massaging each muscle group on both sides of the body. As the client stretches and relaxes, the muscles tend to soften making it easy for them to be massaged deeply. The therapist may use hands, fingers, forearms or elbows to penetrate layers as deep as possible or required, on each side of the body at the same time.

Passive Motion

Passive Motion is more relaxing for the client but shares similar characteristics with the active motion technique. The difference here is that it is the therapist who moves the parts of the body while simultaneously massaging with one hand and moving the body parts with the other. Although this technique is more relaxing for the client, it is quite the taxing task for a single therapist.

Static Pressure

This technique aims at specific areas on which the therapist may use fingers, thumbs or elbows to work on the muscles at a very slow pace. This slow movement allows the muscles to relax, which in return enable the therapist to easily penetrate them. This is a very slow procedure and one muscle can take as long as 20 minutes for it to be massaged sufficiently. The other downside to this type of manipulation is that the recipient can have major discomforts during the process and develop some bruises due to the length of time the muscles are susceptible to pressure. This may become painful especially if you are a beginner so do not hesitate to alert your therapist about any discomforts you may feel immediately.

Negative Pressure

Negative pressure is also known as massage cupping or cupping therapy. This technique uses suction cups placed on the muscles to allow the muscle fibers to expand and spread across in order to release the toxins held up in the tissues. This method is typically faster than other traditional therapeutic massages and techniques. The muscles expand and release lactic acid which then flows through the newly reopened pathways within the body and is later flushed from the tissues along with other toxins. The suction cups encourage the flow of waste fluids which carry the toxins to the body's excretion organs. Lactic acid builds up in the tissues which have been knotted by the tension and normal massage cannot eliminate it. This is why the recipient needs deep tissue massage to unknot the muscles and eliminate lactic acid entirely.

Muscle Stripping

Muscle Stripping is divided into two parts, slow muscle stripping and rapid muscle stripping. Out of all the deep tissue massage techniques, this is the most painful, yet the most effective for those who have had untreated previous injuries for some time and those with chronic pain as a result of incorrect healing.

•Slow Muscle Stripping involves the use of thumbs and/or elbows to make slow but firm and deep massage movements on the muscles.

•Rapid Muscle Stripping should rarely be used unless rapid results are required. When it is used, the recipient makes rapid stretching movements while breathing deeply and the therapist makes rapid and firm movements on the muscles using knuckles and/or elbows. This should only be used in extreme cases.

A full body deep tissue massage may be performed throughout the course of several days while working on each muscle group at a particular time. If you are a beginner, the toxins released may overwhelm you if it is done within one day hence spreading out the treatment appointments over a period of time may be more beneficial in this situation. Plan with your therapist about which specific areas should be addressed and work together for long-lasting effects. Feeling some level of discomfort is normal during and after the massage, however if the discomfort turns into pain you should consult with your therapist. If you still feel sore and bruised after the massage which is beyond your comfort level, consult your physician.

People have different pain tolerance levels and whatever may be painful for you may not be for someone else. Your body may be unable to bear the deep pressure exerted on the deep layers of muscles and soft tissues which allows for the body's natural reflex action which is to resist the massage. Therapists should always work with the clients to know their comfort and pain tolerance levels.

Cost of Therapy

The cost of therapy depends on where you are getting it from, the specific areas you want to be massaged for and the duration of time required. Therapy can be concentrated in certain areas or a full-body massage which can take several days to accomplish may be administered. Massage fees may be set as a flat rate in membership clubs or by the length of the appointment. The sessions can range from 30, 45, 60 or 90 minutes each although longer sessions may also be available. You can get deep tissue massage in specialty clinics, gyms or spas. Hotels and resort spas may be more expensive but it depends on which geographic location you are in to get the service.

You can get the service for as little as $30 or as high as $200 or more, per session. Some places may even have special promotional offers for spouses and friends or groups.

The average cost is usually:

- 30 minutes $30 to $55

- 45 minutes $72

- 60 minutes $85

- 90 minutes $130

You will need to arrive for the session a few minutes earlier so you can relax. A sheet or towel will be used to cover the areas that are not due for massage. Massage oils may be used while some therapists finish off with lotion to moisturize the skin. Some clients prefer soft music to be played, others prefer a quiet environment while some like to have conversations with their spouse, friends or the therapist.

CHAPTER SIX

Pros and Cons Compared to Other Massage Therapies

For you to have a long-term treatment plan you need to weigh the pros and cons of deep tissue massage therapy in comparison to other massage therapies. There are many different types of massage therapies which include deep tissue massage, Swedish massage, sports massage, prenatal massage, reflexology massage and trigger point therapy among many others.

Pros

The massage releases tension, pain, inflammation and lactic acid as well as other toxins trapped within the tissue.

Chronic Pain Relief and Stress Relief

One of the main advantages of having deep tissue massage is the pain relief it brings to you. You may have suffered for many years from chronic pain that has refused to go away despite exercise, medications and other types of therapies. The pain may be due to whiplash, osteoarthritis or other conditions. Deep soft tissues hold toxins that the normal body systems are unable to eliminate. This type of therapy offers you hope and provides you with results so you can overcome these challenges.

You can have therapy after workouts, walking, running, hiking or bodybuilding and general activeness. Stress and tension can also arise from leisure activities such as exercises, gardening or sports. Some careers involving driving, typing, working manually, repetitive work or using hand-held vibrating machines can cause postural imbalances.

Many people agree that deep tissue massage is more effective in relieving osteoarthritis pain compared to other options such as diet, prescriptions medications, OCTs, physical therapy, exercise, and acupuncture and chiropractic therapy. People with fibromyalgia also notice ease in movement and an increased overall range of motion after having a deep tissue massage.

Massage therapists who give deep tissue massage can use hands, fingertips, thumbs, elbows, knuckles and forearms. You can breathe in deeply if you feel slight pain when the tension is being released. Communication between the massage therapist and client is vital. You should convey your level of comfort throughout the treatment to ensure you are receiving the optimal results and not having too much or too little pressure.

Improves Condition of the Muscles

Muscles can form bands and adhesions which make flexibility and mobility difficult. They may crisscross joints making it hard to move the muscles or joints. Professional therapists know how to work on the different layers of muscles including the body's soft tissues found deep beneath the skin. They massage the muscles and the fascia which may have tightened as a result of illness, injury or immobility for a long time. When the fascia is tight or stiff, it allows for the muscles, joints and bones to stiffen but massaging aids in increasing flexibility and mobility when it is administered by a professional therapist.

Treats Chronic Conditions

People with chronic conditions such as osteoarthritis, tennis elbow, carpal tunnel syndrome and fibromyalgia benefit tremendously from deep tissue massage. This is used to relieve the pain and discomfort caused by these conditions. The tissue bands and adhesions that hold the muscles and joints are broken down, increasing range of movement in such conditions.

The main purpose of massage is relaxation, health and wellness. Deep tissue massage can-at times-be used to help the client to relax, however they may not feel relaxed right away but after a few days you start feeling the effects kick in.

Cons

Deep tissue massaging, even when done by a professional can result in some side effects.

•Mild pain

•Discomfort

•Redness

•Swelling

•Muscle stiffness, tenderness and soreness

•Allergic reactions to oils, gels or lotions used

These side effects can arise after deep tissue massage therapy even when it is professionally administered but they usually decrease within one or two days and should eventually go away totally.

If you get these side effects do not blame it on the therapist because this may be normal and this may have been the result even in the most ideal conditions. You may apply ice to the affected area for relief but you should enquire from your massage therapist first. Fortunately, the side effects are mild and you will feel better when they subside and will certainly feel much better than before you ever got such a treatment.

Intuitive

This massage therapy can exceed the limits of the clients' comfort zone causing the muscles to tighten and become tense. This may cause pain and tension which is counter-productive. There may be times that deep tissue massage may generate some degree of pain and discomfort. You should therefore alert the therapist if this happens during your session, even if it's mild. Definitely let the massage therapist know when the pain and soreness is beyond your comfort zone.

CHAPTER SEVEN

Treatment Options

Deep tissue massage is recommended by many doctors all over the world as a treatment option for many ailments and diseases. It uses systematic techniques consisting of using deep, slow and firm strokes. Within the scope of deep tissue massage therapy, there are different treatment options. Many people prefer this massage because it has no adverse side effects except the mild ones which typically go away within 1-3 days.

You have a choice among the many different treatment options which include:

•Deep tissue massage

•Swedish massage

•Sports massage

•Prenatal massage

•Trigger point massage

•Reflexology massage

•Hot stone massage

•Aromatherapy

Each of these treatments have their own benefits, pros and cons. Furthermore, each treatment is meant for certain purposes so you should discuss with your therapist to understand what the best option is for you.

Precautions

Although massage is therapeutic, it may not be appropriate for people who have the following conditions:

•Skin rashes

•Burns

•Open and unhealed wounds

•Infectious skin diseases

•Recent fractures

•Heart disease

•Pregnancy unless recommended by the doctor

•Deep venous thrombosis (DVT) and other blood disorders

•Severe osteoporosis

You should not have a deep tissue massage:

•Immediately after surgery

•After chemotherapy or radiation, unless the doctor recommends

•If you are prone to blood clots or you are on blood thinning medications

•Heart disease

•Pregnant unless it is administered by a massage therapist specializing in pregnancy

No massage should be done over open wounds, bruises, inflamed skin, hernia, tumors or recently fractured areas. If you have severe osteoporosis, you should consult your doctor before receiving deep tissue massage.

•Avoid eating a heavy meal before having deep tissue massage.

•You need to rest and relax before and after the treatment.

•Consume plenty of water and or herbal teas. This will help to eliminate metabolic waste products from the body.

•Stretch yourself after the massage to enhance and aid the recovery process.

Deep tissue massage is done professionally so it is unlikely that you will be able to do it on your own. Furthermore, it would be difficult for you to reach certain areas of your body. To have it done effectively, you need a certified massage therapist who is competent and has the right knowledge, training and experience in this field. However, self-administered massage within certain areas is possible such as elbows, fingers, arms, neck, legs, feet, toes, hamstrings and others body parts however, perform and your own risk.

CHAPTER EIGHT

Before and After Results

The before and after results of massage depends on the individual, since everyone is different. The massage is customized to the client's needs. People who complain of neck stiffness, sore/heavy shoulders, lower back pain, upper back pain, shortened hamstrings, stiff or uneven hips, painful elbows and forearms can all benefit from this therapy and help correct these problems. You can minimize the exposure in the first place to such conditions by sitting in the ergonomically correct position on the chair at the desk if you are a secretary, IT personnel or if you are a driver. Stretch from time to time, get training for proper lifting, pushing and pulling techniques for heavy loads. Wearing health bracelets helps to aid in relaxation if you are a busy executive.

When someone receives deep tissue massage, they may feel mild pain and soreness to the areas massaged however, in the long run you will feel rejuvenated and happy that the toxins previously held up in the tissues are released. Although there may be times that the massage is not pleasant, after several sessions the pain subsides and you have more flexibility while the posture is corrected increasing your mobility when the fascia and deep layers of tissues are worked on using the therapeutic principles.

The pain should be bearable and you should feel better afterwards. However, the massage does not have to hurt, your therapist should try to make it as comfortable as reasonably possible for you. You don't have to bite your lips, grip the towel with pain or yell. Focusing on deep breathing is all that you need.

There are people who believe that in order to be beneficial, deep tissue massage has to be painful. This is negative thinking. In fact, this type of therapy can be very relaxing. The muscles and soft tissues can be manipulated in a way that is not painful to the recipient, yet still effective. The top muscles can be warmed and stroked slowly to allow the therapist to reach and work on the deep layers of the muscles and the soft tissues. This has to be done in a way that the muscles do not subconsciously tense up, further resisting their accessibility.

Our bodies react to pain naturally. The body's natural reflex action of tightening up under discomfort can make the muscles resist the massage if they experience pain. The therapist may use several treatment options to get the desired results. The after results may not be noticeable right away or all the time but most people say they feel great afterwards-certainly much better than before getting the massage. Although some people enjoy the deep pressure others prefer a gentle touch. Deep tissue massage can be combined with other relaxation massages such as Swedish massage to get clients to relax and loosen up. It is advisable that you rest and relax after the massage especially for the first day. Some people feel sleepy as the kidneys and skin work to eliminate the toxins released during deep tissue massage, however it is advised that they try to stay awake to aid the therapist during the massaging process.

CHAPTER NINE

The Final Verdict

Deep tissue massage is used to heal and recuperate the muscles and rejuvenate your body by allowing therapists to get to the core of the muscles. The deep tissue therapist works on the structure of the muscles to increase their elasticity, flexibility and help them release tension for optimum performance and to get the muscles healthy again. Some clients have pain and soreness after deep tissue massage therapy but this should subside within a day or so. People feel relaxed and re-energized after a few days of experiencing the optimum benefits of this therapy. You should take a warm bath after treatment, drink plenty of water and herbal teas to help in the elimination process of the toxins as you relax and take time to rest.

There are many do it yourself therapies available if you truly want to experience something you can do on your own before you think about professional treatment options. Reflexology is also another great alternative medicine which focuses on the body's natural ability to heal itself through therapeutic means by targeting reflex points in the hands, feet and ears to stimulate all internal organs, glands bones and joints to restore your body's natural balance. Check out the book, *"Holistic Reflexology Guide: Alternative Medicine for a Happier, Healthier and Healthier You"*. This book provides you with a different perspective on dealing with the struggles of your life-exclusively through the art of reflexology. What reflexology allows for is a bonding of the mind, body and spirit to alleviate the external struggles of life by manipulating that energy into a self-healing internal process-this may sound similar to meditation but is completely different and a purely natural remedy. The book provides you with a simple look into reflexology-after all, reflexology itself deals with simplifying your pains through deep relaxation of the mind, body and spirit. The content of this book touches on a little bit about a lot of things reflexology related. By simplifying key concepts, the essence of the main message gets across while keeping the jargoning to a minimum. Hopefully I've some put things into perspective and got you thinking about investing your time into this book. The decision to purchase is ultimately your-no pressure. More info available at my author's page, amazon.com/author/m.s.d.

Author's Note

Throughout this read if you have gained any form of value at all, please take a moment out of your invaluable time to rate this book. Catering to the specific needs of individuals in terms of providing the audience with valuable content can sometimes be a daunting task from the author's perspective since peoples' preferences vary greatly.

Providing your honest feedback in terms of a brief review can greatly help us independent authors to determine the usefulness of the content and find ways to better deliver customer oriented information. We rely on fair reviews to continue to make a name for ourselves and build a brand around our publications.

Your honest feedback is profoundly appreciated. Thank you for purchasing this e-book. Hopefully the time and money you've invested in this book has paid off!